Loving Me, Myself and "Her:" Through Perimenopause and Beyond

By Dr. Joy'El Ballard

Jive for today
Laugh often
Love yourself

Dr. Jy'El

TABLE OF CONTENTS

ACKNOWLEDGMENTS

This book is my expression of love for my patients and all women who are discovering their potential and making it a reality.

My sincere gratitude to the beautiful women who are my cheering squad daily, my mother and my sisters in addition to my children- Jocelyn, Symone and Justin who inspire me to be the best version of myself. I would like to thank my father who has always saw my potential before I can even realize it in all my endeavors. I would like to thank my brothers for their love and support.

I am most grateful for the encouragement and love from my husband, Corey, who reminds me that true love exists.

INTRODUCTION

Menopause is not for sissies!! Your mom may have sat you down to have the "sex talk" while you were a teenager. But did she sit you down to have the "menopause talk" since you've been an adult? She didn't? Well, menopause isn't usually a common topic of discussion, most likely because a lot of women experience several changes that they would like to forget during menopause or the menopausal transition – unpleasant changes that a lot of women would like to suppress. You may have heard your mom complain about hot flashes or what some may call "personal summers", but she didn't warn you, did she? Most women are unaware of what those are until it hits them in the face...literally. A sudden sensation of extreme heat in the upper body, particularly the face, neck and chest that can be overwhelming and embarrassing!

Dramatic changes in your menstrual cycle, mood swings, mental fog, trouble sleeping, weight gain, vaginal dryness and decreased libido – so much to look forward to! Your significant other may advise you to see a doctor, because you are not acting "normal". Well guess what? These changes are normal even though it doesn't feel "normal" at all. It can feel like a roller coaster that you can't get off of. Welcome to perimenopause and the next stop – menopause!

Night sweats, mood irritability, facial acne and high blood pressure is how it started for me. On one hand, I felt like a teenager again worrying about what I look like, then on the other hand, I felt old, because I was struggling to keep my blood pressure down. And this all started at 39! "I'm too young for this!" I told myself. So many things swirl in your head as you approach 40. You wonder if you've accomplished what you've wanted to accomplish so far. You check off goals that you know you wanted to achieve. But then you get to a point and wonder if there's more that you need to do. And maybe my daddy sensed that I was comfortable in the moment, so he told me, "But you're not done yet." I didn't really consider this possibility the first few times he said it, but when I turned 40, a light bulb switched on and I thought "I CAN do more." So, then I had to figure out what "more" meant, while my body was experiencing changes that were unexpected and uncontrollable.

For me, "more" was helping women through this journey of perimenopause and menopause. I've had so many women visit my office who were wondering what's going on with their bodies and their minds, feeling lost and blindsided and asking me, "What can I read to get more information?" I had another light bulb moment! I'd write a guide for women about what to expect during menopause. I also wanted to include some positive affirmations to help women through "the change" and make sure that in the process, they'd show themselves some love; thus, the title *Loving Me, Myself and "Her"*. That means loving the skin that you're in despite the creepy crawler sensations you feel when you experience different symptoms throughout the process. It's about loving yourself AND your vagina. The "Her." Let's face it, if your vagina is not happy, you're not happy. So, we gotta show her some love too. I'll talk about how later.

So, the principles of Loving Me, Myself and "Her" are:

- Loving Me is defined by loving who you are. The person you look at in the mirror every day.
- Loving Myself is defined by loving what I stand for and what I am becoming.
- Loving "Her" is simply showing love and respect for your vagina.
- LOVE YOURSELF through it all; The glowing beads of sweat, the love handles and the vagina that needs extra loving!

Let's turn this "menopause takeover" into a menopause makeover! So, let's get started!

1: MENOPAUSE OR PERIMENOPAUSE: THAT IS THE QUESTION!

Let's start with some definitions. Many women don't know the difference between perimenopause or the "menopausal transition" and menopause. So, I'll say get ready for a change! Now change can be a good thing even when it's uncomfortable. If you accept it and maneuver your way through it, you'll be fine!

Perimenopause is the years of transition from the reproductive years to the non-reproductive years in a woman's life. It can start as early as age 39 and anywhere between two to ten years prior to menopause. Your hormones, specifically estrogen, will fluctuate for days, weeks and even months. Your estrogen levels, specifically estradiol, can increase, decrease or remain normal and your progesterone levels can decrease or remain normal.

Menopause is the permanent cessation of menstrual cycles. No bleeding of any type for 12 consecutive months. The average age is 51. By this time, estrogen and progesterone are both on a steady decline. Testosterone and Dehydroepiandrosterone (DHEA) both decline with age, but at a much slower rate than estrogen. Premature menopause occurs before the age of 40 and early menopause occurs between the ages of 40 and 45.

Postmenopause is the time after the onset of menopause.

There are some women who barely notice this milestone of aging. Lucky them! My mom breezed through menopause without a symptom. I started experiencing night sweats at age 39! Lucky me!! More of us notice a significant change in our physical, psychological and emotional selves. Sometimes we don't even recognize ourselves. We think, who is this woman? This can be scary and disheartening! But again, the key here is knowing what to expect, so at least you won't be thrown off guard. This is a natural process that every woman will experience, which can be a smooth or very bumpy ride. Again, this is NATURAL, although it may not feel natural at all. In your journey, embrace what's coming your way and push through it by being well informed. Develop a strategy with your healthcare provider to handle YOUR experience of menopause. It can be totally different for your mother, sister or your friend, so don't compare yourself to others.

Words of Affirmation:

Learning never stops and change is constant. So, I will learn to step out of the box, out of my comfort zone and CHANGE.

2: TALK IT OUT!

Now let's discuss some common questions and answers:

"Why don't women talk about menopause more often?"

Being embarrassed, confused and isolated are some reasons why women don't talk about menopause.

"Aren't I too young to be going through these changes?"

No. Unfortunately, some women begin the transition before they reach 40 and some much later than that. It is different for every woman.

"Am I the only one going through this, because none of my friends have mentioned it?"

No, they haven't mentioned it, because they are thinking the same thing!!

As a 40-something year old woman, I have had similar thoughts myself. Some women are in DENIAL. A patient of mine said, "If I admit to these symptoms, then I'll be considered old." This patient was only 53 years old! She then asked me, "You know what age those senior living places start accepting residents?" She answered her own question and said, "55! Society is already assuming I'm old at the age of 55. And that is depressing!"

Or, imagine going out with your girlfriends and you suddenly say, "My vagina has been so dry, how's yours?" What a buzz killer! In the face of all these feelings, you must aim to educate yourself through this natural process. You can get a sense of what to expect and what your options are to treat certain symptoms of menopause. "Dr. Google" is not always accurate, which is why I wrote this book. Dr. Google may be able to give you an outline of what to expect in menopause and/or scare you half to death, but a practicing physician will be able to give more detail and current recommendations on menopausal treatment.

You need to talk to someone about what you are experiencing. You may feel that you are the ONLY one going through these changes, but you must know that you ARE NOT ALONE! I encourage you to talk to your gynecologist or primary care physician. I know sometimes it may be an uncomfortable conversation, but it must happen. It is important to have a good relationship with your physician, because if you don't and you're not able to reveal your symptoms, then you are missing out on potential options that may help you. So, if you don't have a physician that makes you feel comfortable about discussing personal changes, then you may want to consider switching to another physician who may make this experience less awkward. You need to have an honest conversation, so that you can be better served through this process. When you find a physician that suits your needs, make an appointment just to talk. You don't have to wait until your next annual exam, because quite honestly, that may not be enough time. It's difficult to fit the spectrum of menopause into a 15 minute well woman appointment. Believe me, I know! As a physician, 15 minutes goes fast! Write down your questions and concerns. Make sure your physician is aware of your medical conditions and all of the medications that you are taking, as well as, your family history that may have an impact on your options. This information certainly drives the conversation about certain symptoms as well as treatment options. For example, there could be a medication that you're taking that is causing a symptom of menopause.

In my office: A 40-year-old comes in complaining about five months of decreased libido. While obtaining a full history, she revealed that she started Prozac for depression six months ago. Jackpot! Certain antidepressants can decrease your libido.

Do NOT suffer in silence!

Please talk to your friend, your sister or even your mother about their menopausal experiences! Now, take it easy on your mother if she hasn't already told you a thing or two about menopause. She may have been embarrassed about what she went through or she may have just breezed through it without any issues (lucky gal!). But it is good just to have someone you can talk to about your symptoms and just to share information with. And don't forget to talk to your daughters. Give them a heads up about menopause. They will appreciate it when they get to be our age.

More importantly, talk to your significant other because this affects them too. Communication is so essential in a healthy relationship, especially when major changes are occurring. And this is MAJOR. Your mind and body are doing things beyond your control. So, after speaking with your physician and getting more information about what's going on and why, you can share this information with your significant other. I frequently tell my perimenopausal and menopausal patients, "Now go home and tell your partner that this is not your fault...this is NATURAL." This also lifts some of the burden off of your partner because there are times when your partner will blame themselves about certain issues, i.e. decreased libido.

Communicating the natural processes of perimenopause/menopause can give your loved ones some sense of understanding and empathy, hopefully. Revealing your journey and communicating your realities can be liberating. So, try it! Be open and welcoming to anticipatory change. Change can be a good thing.

Words of Affirmation:

I will love myself enough to voice my feelings and concerns without fear of judgment or embarrassment. I am not OLD, just more experienced! I will LOVE me for what I am becoming.

3: WHAT IN THE BLOODY HELL?!

In my office: A 45-year-old woman states her periods have been very heavy over the last six months. She reports she wears a super tampon and a pad at the same time. She is afraid to leave her house during this time, because she is afraid of having an accident in her clothing.

In my office: A 42-year-old woman comes in stating her periods are all over the place for the last six months. One month, she had her period twice. She had skipped her period for two months, so she took three pregnancy tests, which were negative. She had no idea why this was happening because in her words, "It can't be menopause, because I'm too young for that!"

One of the first signs of perimenopause is a change in your menstrual cycle. Your cycle can be heavier and/or longer, it can be lighter and/or shorter. It can occur twice in one month or you may skip a month or two. They can become more painful or you could have worsening premenstrual symptoms (PMS). Abnormal bleeding after the age of 35 usually requires a work-up that may include a pelvic sonogram, a biopsy from the uterine lining and possibly some blood work. Typically, after eliminating other factors that may cause irregular bleeding after 40 – stress, pregnancy, thyroid disorder, uterine fibroids, polyps or certain medications – perimenopause is most likely the culprit. Many women believe that any symptom of menopause doesn't appear until closer to age 50. So they automatically think that something is wrong since they feel too young for menopause. This is simply not true. As I stated before, you can start to have symptoms as early as age 39.

In my office: A 44-year-old who is having irregular periods and some hot flashes, but she is mostly bothered by her periods that she can't predict. She stopped her birth control pills about 5 years ago since her husband got a vasectomy. After discussing her medical history, *which was essentially uncomplicated, I suggested that she restart the pill. Her response, "I thought I was too old to take birth control pills."*

This is a common response when birth control pills are suggested after the age of 40. I must tell you that it is SAFE to go on a birth control pill if you don't have any contraindications to hormones. Contraindications to taking hormones are being a smoker, history of blood clots in the deep veins of the leg or lungs, history of migraines with aura, history of poorly controlled high blood pressure or history of breast cancer. If you are not a candidate for birth control pills or you simply don't want to take them, then your alternatives to managing heavy menstrual cycles are a Mirena Intrauterine Device (IUD) or a procedure called a uterine ablation. A hysterectomy, which is the removal of your uterus and cervix, would be definitive treatment and should be a shared decision between you and your healthcare provider. Or you don't have to do anything and can simply monitor your cycles. However, if your cycles are causing you to become anemic, then I suggest you do something about it.

I inform my patients that many women go back on the pill to help them transition into menopause. Usually, I recommend a low-dose birth control pill to my patients in their early to mid-40s. Low dose means less hormones, but the pills are still effective and hopefully have fewer side effects. This can address the menstrual irregularities, as well as some hot flashes, and many women are happy with this choice. But again, discuss your medical history and options with your healthcare provider to see if this is a good choice for you. Your healthcare provider can review the risks and benefits of starting a birth control pill, then you can decide if taking the pill is right for you. Hormone replacement therapy (HRT) may be offered if you're going through these changes closer to the age of 50.

You may wonder if going on the pill would stop you from going into menopause – NOPE! Taking them just adds back hormones to better control your symptoms, but naturally the amount of estrogen being produced will continue to decline. Now you can't stay on the birth control forever, although some may wish they could. Studies show that you can safely continue taking the pill up until you're 50-55. When you stop and continue to have significant menopausal symptoms, then you can switch to HRT which is at even a lower dose.

So, what about checking hormones? A lot of women come in asking me to check their hormones to see if they are going through menopause. Guess what? This is not the standard of care nor even necessary in most cases. If your periods are skipping months and you're having hot flashes, then you're likely perimenopausal after excluding other possibilities. During perimenopause, your hormones can be in the normal range at different times, because hormones are fluctuating throughout the day and on a daily basis. Follicle-stimulating hormone, or FSH, is the hormone secreted by your ovaries that increases while estrogen decreases, as you approach menopause. This value will be variable, especially in perimenopause. Your FSH can be in the normal range, but you can still be perimenopausal.

So, checking your FSH isn't really going to give me any extra information, which is why I go by your symptomatology. Checking hormones may be helpful if I suspect a thyroid disorder, then I would check your thyroid hormone levels. There are circumstances that would prompt me to check your FSH level, such as women who have had an ablation, a Mirena IUD or a hysterectomy. All of these could cause your menstrual cycles to cease or be totally eliminated with a hysterectomy. Since the cessation of menstrual cycles for 12 months defines menopause, it would be difficult to determine if you've had one of these procedures, then I would consider checking your FSH level based on other symptoms.

Essentially, your estrogen is currently on a roller coaster ride that you can't stop. So, buckle your seat belt and hold on! It will eventually slow down, then gradually stop and you will enter a new journey of freedom from worrying about ruining a pretty pair of panties.

Words of Affirmation:

I will continue to love me despite the uncomfortable changes I may endure.

4: HOT & SEXY? NO. HOT & BOTHERED!

In my office: A 49-year-old woman with mostly regular cycles (she skipped one month and thought it was due to stress) came in reporting frequent hot flashes that were disturbing her at work and at home.

The sudden sensation of extreme heat in the upper body is called a hot flush. But most of us call it hot flashes! If it occurs during nighttime sleep, we call them night sweats. Your experiences may be something like:

- In a meeting, suddenly your chest, neck and face turn beet red.
- Sitting at your desk, your coworker notices beads of sweat on your forehead.
- Sleeping in bed, you wake up drenched in sweat thinking did I pee in the bed?! (I experienced this thought myself!)

Does any of this sound familiar? These are all examples of vasomotor symptoms that occur with perimenopause and/or menopause triggered by small elevations in core body temperature. About 50-82% of U.S. women who experience natural menopause report these symptoms. These episodes can last one to five minutes. They vary in frequency and duration. 87% of women report having hot flashes daily. However, there may be some who experience them two to three times per week. Vasomotor symptoms can be associated with perspiration, flushing, chills, clamminess, anxiety and occasionally heart palpitations. Severe vasomotor symptoms occur more frequently, up to every hour and can be very bothersome. Women with severe vasomotor symptoms may experience diminished quality of sleep, difficulty concentrating and irritability.

My patients almost always ask, "So when do they stop?" And I answer, "I have no idea!" Sorry, I know you were expecting a better answer. The truth is that it is so variable, that the overall duration of hot flashes remains unclear. Prior reports estimated they can last anywhere from six months to two years. Now, the average duration could be between four to ten years. Unfortunately for some, it could be longer than 10 years or indefinitely. But there is hope in that they do decrease in frequency and intensity later on in postmenopause. Hopefully, you won't need that portable fan forever!

As women, we like to look and feel sexy. Water dripping from your hair when you didn't just get out of a pool or wet spots on your blouse is NOT sexy, right? So, we have to move toward getting our sexy back amid hot flashes. I like to start by giving the following recommendations that patients can do on their own:

- First, invest in a portable fan (I am not kidding). Just periodically pretend you're auditioning for your favorite performer on stage and they require your hair to blow in the wind like Beyoncé.
- Dress in layers. A cute camisole or tank dress with a cute blazer or cardigan that you can take off and on will help.

- If you have mostly night sweats, then wear short pajamas or nothing at all!
- Avoid triggers. Some of us realize that our flashes occur after drinking caffeine or wine or eating spicy food. Now I'm not saying you must give up wine, but you may just have to enjoy it in the privacy of your own home.
- Also, rooms that are too hot can also trigger hot flashes. If you're interested in moving to Alaska, this may be the way to go. But the rest of us can just lower the room temperature at home or in the workplace. Our family or coworkers may not like it, but they can easily put on a sweatshirt or a sweater.
  - If you are a smoker, STOP SMOKING!
  - And STRESS can certainly contribute to the occurrence of hot flashes or night sweats. You must manage your stress level. Easy, right? Nope!

The average adult human body is composed of about 50-65% water. As women, we feel like our bodies are 20% water and 80% stress! We can be pulled in so many directions – wife, mother, professional, daughter, sister and friend and have the guilt that we must be great at EVERYTHING! This is stressful! And while we're fulfilling all these roles, our bodies go through some twists and turns we weren't expecting. So, once we convince ourselves that we don't have to do it ALL, we make time to take care of our bodies by giving them the appropriate attention.

In my office: The same patient states she dresses in layers and keeps the temperature at 65 degrees at home, but still is uncomfortable with these flashes.

So, what are other options? Estrogen is the first Food and Drug Administration (FDA) approved treatment for hot flashes and is 90% effective. Over the past 50 years, there has been variable enthusiasm for HRT during menopause. Initially, it was the best thing since sliced bread. Then after more studies, people avoided it like the plague. Most recently, studies recommend using the lowest effective dose for the shortest amount of time for treatment of menopausal symptoms.

The Women's Health Initiative (WHI) was launched in the early 1990s to study hormone treatment for menopause and its effects. The risks and benefits continue to be examined. Based on varying results, different healthcare providers may have differing opinions about starting their patients on hormones. It is important for you to be aware of your options, so that you can make an informed decision about this potential treatment.

There are different modes of delivery of hormones to improve your vasomotor symptoms. There are pills, transdermal patches and gels, including the following:

- Estrogen gels – Divigel or Elestrin
- Estrogen patches – Vivelle, Vivelle Dot or Climara
- Estrogen spray – Evamist

There are other methods that address the vaginal symptoms of menopause and I'll discuss that in Chapter 7.

If you still have a uterus, you CANNOT take Estrogen alone. Estrogen alone can stimulate an increase in cells of the lining of your uterus, which can lead to uterine cancer over time. Therefore, adding progesterone is necessary to counteract this effect. You have the option of taking estrogen and progesterone separately by taking estrogen daily, then taking progesterone continuously or cyclically for 12-14 days of the month. Or you can take a formulation that contains both, such as Activella, Angeliq or Combipatch. Duavee is a newer medication that is useful for women with hot flashes and who are also at risk for osteoporosis, which is bone loss. Discuss with your healthcare provider which medication and method is appropriate for you.

Hormone replacement pills are taken orally daily. There are skin patches that you can change weekly or twice a week, depending on which one you have. There is also gels that you rub on your forearm or upper thigh daily or biweekly, depending on which one you have. I recommend that with any regimen, you start with the lowest dose first, then work your way up if you need to. Please have realistic goals. You should aim for something that lessens your symptoms and allows you to function day-to-day. If you aim for something that will totally eliminate your symptoms, you may be disappointed. Be aware that it can take any of these methods about two to four weeks to notice an improvement. Sorry, nothing works overnight. So give it a good try.

Do I need to check your hormones after starting HRT? No, studies show there are few indications for the measurement of hormone levels to determine success of therapy if you are on HRT. Typically, success of therapy is determined by the improvement of your symptoms. There are cases where I may recommend checking your hormones and that is when a patient is on testosterone therapy. Testosterone levels need to be monitored initially to ensure that it is in an appropriate range for a woman.

Some might ask, "Well how long can you stay on HRT?" Recent studies recommend that you stop HRT after 10 years of use. Taking it longer may increase your risk of breast cancer, blood clots in deep veins and heart disease.

But what about my 70-year-old grandmother who is still on hormones? Yes, there are some women who try to wean themselves off of them, but still have symptoms that affect their daily living. So, they feel their quality of life is more important and they continue hormones despite the possible risks. But this is what an informed decision is. You learn about your options and consider the risks, then decide if you want to move forward with it. And that's okay!

Now what are Bioidentical hormones? At one point every patient was coming in asking for bioidentical hormones, because they heard that they are so much "better" than the standard HRT. Bioidentical hormones are plant-derived hormones that are chemically similar to your natural hormones that are produced by the body. Synthetic hormones have a different chemical structure and may not have the same effects on target tissues as natural hormones. So, you may ask, how do I know which hormone is bioidentical? Estrogen and progesterone are the two hormones we typically try to replace in menopause. So, examples of bioidentical estrogen are Estradiol or Estrace. Prometrium is an example of a bioidentical progesterone.

Compounded bioidentical hormones are hormones that are made by compounding pharmacists and available in various forms – oral, sublingual, transdermal gels, implants and suppositories. Some physicians may prescribe a compounded form of hormones to address your symptoms. Be aware that compounded formulations are not FDA approved and possibly unregulated so you could get too much or too little of what you actually need. Be aware that varying ingredients and preservatives are used in addition to the actual hormone to make this compounded product. This can make it difficult to identify the etiology of adverse effects if it is difficult to identify the active ingredient within the compounded formula. Now I'm not saying that you should avoid this option, but just be informed and know what you are getting. Knowing a good compounding pharmacy is important.

Again, I am writing this to educate you on all of the possibilities. Talk to your healthcare provider to discuss your options and which may be a good fit for your life. Also, be aware of some of the side effects if you choose to take hormones, including breast tenderness, bloating, headaches and abnormal vaginal bleeding. Now, for those of you who can't take hormones, like breast cancer survivors, or who just want to avoid it all together, I've dedicated the next two chapters to you.

Perimenopause or menopause can vary from woman to woman and this is true for treatment. One treatment may work well for your sister but may not be a good fit for you. Embrace your uniqueness and your new normal!

Words of Affirmation:

I love myself, because my sexy exudes from within, not my outward appearance.

Dr. Joy'El Ballard

5: YOU WANNA SAY NO TO HORMONES? HERE ARE SOME ALTERNATIVES

Some women just don't want hormones and that's okay. It's your body and this is your decision. No one knows you better than yourself. Some women don't have a choice, due to certain medical conditions, like a history of breast cancer, specifically hormone-sensitive breast cancer or any other type of hormone-sensitive cancer, blood clots in deep veins of their body such as the leg or lungs, migraines with aura, uncontrolled high blood pressure, heart disease or active liver disease.

Personally, I am a fan of trying the "natural" options first. Taking hormones is not a requirement. Start with the basics – eating healthy and exercise! You are what you eat, so eat the rainbow!! As I stated in the previous chapter, you may recognize certain foods or drinks trigger menopausal vasomotor symptoms, so avoid those. Your daily goal for your diet should be 35 g of fiber, 8-12 servings of fruits and vegetables, good fats like avocados and nuts and healthier proteins like grass-fed meats and beans. Phytoestrogens or soy isoflavones are plant-derived substances that act like biologic estrogen. However, given its estrogenic effects, should be avoided in women with a history of hormone-sensitive cancers. Omega-3 fatty acids are good, because they have an anti-inflammatory action that positively affects cells in the brain, heart and bone. You can find them in spinach, kale and fish. The omega-3 fatty acids that make up fish oil tablets are Eicosapentaenoic acid (EPA) and Docosahexaenoic (DHA). The recommendation is one to three grams per day.

Exercise is ALWAYS a must! Keep your body moving, because it releases endorphins, which improve your natural immunity, as well as, reduce stress. Menopause is like a form of internal stress within your body. Aim to exercise four to five days per week for at least thirty minutes per day.

Relizen is a newer supplement made from a Swedish flower pollen extract that has been shown to decrease the frequency and intensity of hot flashes. Many herbal remedies have been studied in the realm of menopause. None have been proven to definitely work, but small case studies have shown some benefit compared to placebo. Black cohosh is an herb that has been largely studied, however no studies have definitively proven that it improves hot flashes. Some research has reported that it may help some women compared to placebo.

Acupuncture has been investigated as a treatment for hot flashes, but the evidence is limited and it may only cause a slight decrease in the frequency of hot flashes.

Most recently, Cannabidiol (CBD) has been gaining more attention in treating multiple medical conditions. It is a chemical that exists in hemp plants and marijuana. Even though it is a byproduct of marijuana, it is not psychoactive, so does not cause the "high" associated with marijuana. But the legality of it in the U.S. varies from state to state. It is possible that CBD oil could help treat the symptoms of menopause. It can potentially improve mood, sleep and frequency of hot flashes, but this has yet to be proven. I have had a few patients that has tried it and it is working well for them. It may work for some, but not for others. There are a lot more herbs/supplements that I did not mention that some studies suggest may improve menopausal vasomotor symptoms. You could try those too, but again, make sure you discuss this with your physician first.

There are alternative prescribed medications that can improve vasomotor symptoms. There is increasing evidence that the following medications are effective for treatment of vasomotor symptoms associated with menopause:

- Paroxetine (Brisdelle) is a very low dose of the brand name Paxil, which is an antidepressant.
- Venlaxafine (Effexor) is an antianxiety medication that has been shown to improve vasomotor symptoms.
- Clonidine is a medication used for high blood pressure that has been shown to be helpful in treating hot flashes.

- Gabapentin is an anti-seizure medication that seems to help night sweats at its lower doses.

Paroxetine is the only one that is FDA approved. The others are not, but many studies have shown them to work for some women. Gabapentin can be sedating, so I would recommend this to those of you who experience most of your hot flashes at night. But again, a conversation with your doctor is important. Before you start any medication, you must know if it is compatible with the medical conditions that you may have and any other medications you are taking. And you know there are always potential side effects, so keep that in mind too and ask questions. If your hot flashes are mild and you can function with them, then you don't have to take anything. Go on and live your best life with short personal vacays in the tropics!

Words of Affirmation:

I am empowered to know my options and decide what enters my temple – mind, body and soul.

6: BLESS THE SURVIVORS!

Breast cancer is the most common type of invasive disease in American women. The lifetime risk of this disease is one in eight women. I know the diagnosis as well as the treatment of this disease can have deleterious effects and affect how women view themselves. To my breast cancer survivors, I know you have enough on your plate and menopausal symptoms are the least of your worries. The diagnosis of breast cancer is devastating for most and I applaud you for pushing through your journey with strength and positivity. Treatment can include surgery, radiation treatment, chemotherapy and hormonal therapies. So, given these therapies, I know some of you may have been abruptly introduced to menopause during your treatment. The treatment may have been chemotherapy or other medications that suppress your ovaries or significantly reduce the amount of circulating estrogens. Many of you will experience hot flashes, some worse than others, depending on which treatment regimen you have. Unlike women who experience natural menopause, there's no gradual ride uphill and there's no grace period. You just get thrown right into the pot of hot water...literally! Common hormonal therapies are either Tamoxifen, which is usually given to premenopausal women with hormone-sensitive breast cancer, or Arimidex, which is usually given to postmenopausal women.

Those of you who underwent surgeries to remove your ovaries (that may be related to a diagnosis of hormone-sensitive cancer), which places you into surgical menopause, had an abrupt introduction to menopause. Suppressing your ovaries through treatment or taking the ovaries completely away causes menopausal symptoms. If you have hormone-sensitive breast cancer, your physician will likely discuss the risks and benefits of removing your ovaries if you have completed childbearing. But it's good to have a conversation beforehand, whether it's about medical treatment or surgery, to discuss what to expect. You can also discuss your options prior to moving forward with treatment options.

So, for those of you with hormone-sensitive cancer (specific breast cancers, ovarian cancer and uterine cancer), hormonal replacement therapy for vasomotor symptoms is not an option for you. I mentioned non-hormonal options in the prior chapter that may be of benefit to you. But again, discuss your options with your health care provider, including your oncologist. Nutritious diet, regular exercise and managing your stress levels are also crucial in dealing with the effects of conventional treatment of hormone-sensitive cancer.

For your vaginal symptoms, you may use over-the-counter remedies. Some oncologists may allow vaginal estrogen in tablet form (least systemic absorption), only if the natural remedies don't work and if your breast cancer is not hormone-sensitive. This is a conversation that needs to include your oncologist.

This disease can affect so many aspects of your femininity. The surgery alone affects body image, which can subsequently affect sex appeal. Treatment affects vaginal health deleteriously, which can prevent you from enjoying sex. So, let's talk about this in the next two chapters.

Words of Affirmation:

I love ME for my strength and won't allow any diagnosis to dominate my destiny.

7: HELP "HER!" MY VAGINA FEELS LIKE THE SAHARA DESERT!

Don't worry, you're not alone! Vaginal symptoms are the second most common symptom associated with the transition into menopause. Genitourinary syndrome of menopause (GSM) is the newest term used when describing menopausal effects on the labia, vagina, urethra and bladder. Estrogen helps in creating lactobacilli, which are bacteria in the vagina that make glycogen. Glycogen contributes to the alkaline pH of a healthy vagina. Therefore, the loss of estrogen creates an acidic environment in the vagina, which makes it susceptible to irritation and infection. This could also lead to urinary tract infections. The loss of the superficial cells that line the vaginal walls also causes thinning and fragility. Vaginal secretions decrease due to the changes in the blood supply to the vagina. All this defines vaginal atrophy or dryness. The bottom line is your vagina is not like she used to be!

In my office: A 49-year-old woman comes in complaining about on and off vaginal irritation and itching. She denies changes in her soaps or detergents. She has the same sexual partner but is losing interest in sex due to this issue.

This could be a sign of vaginal atrophy - vaginal or vulvar dryness, discharge, itching and painful sex. Sometimes it may feel like you always have a vaginal infection. Or you actually may have a recurrence of vaginal infections due to the changes in the pH of the vagina. Unfortunately, unlike hot flashes that eventually improve over time, these symptoms worsen as menopause ensues. I recommend you address it early on instead of waiting until the camels come home. My second recommendation is to take a handheld mirror and look down there, ladies. Look at your vaginas and labia! Don't be afraid – it's your vagina! It's important to know what changes are occurring down there so you can recognize possible abnormal changes. Well, what can you use for your dry vagina? You have options. And petroleum jelly is NOT one of them.

You can start with over-the-counter options. I advise you to use lubrication during sex at ALL times no matter what. Keep the lube in your nightstand drawer! Even though you may feel like you don't need it, extra lube never hurt anybody. Unless you have a sensitive vagina and are prone to infections, you must be careful about what kind you use. There are different kinds of lubricants, as well as vaginal moisturizers, including, Revaree, Luvena, KY-Silk-E and Replens. You can apply these daily.

Lubricants should be used when engaging in intercourse to reduce friction. You don't want to start any fires! If you don't, you may feel intense burning in your vagina like a fire! Moisturizers can be used on a long-term basis to replace secretions daily.

Some good lubricants to try are:

Water-based	Silicone-based	Oil-based
KY jelly, Just Like Me, Astroglide	Pure Pleasure, Pink	Coconut oil

You can also make your own coconut oil suppository! Get a mini-ice cube tray and fill it with liquified coconut oil and freeze it. When you are about to go to bed, lay a towel down on the bed, get a cube of coconut oil and put it in your vagina. Lay down, go to sleep and let the magical soothing oil do its thing! Remember silicone and oil-based lubricants are not compatible with condoms and some are not compatible with sex toys.

There's also a new pH-balanced option that contains hyaluronic acid (Revaree) that is helpful for moisturizing the vaginal walls. Hyaluronic acid is common in a lot of skin care products due to its hydrating properties. Now it's available for your vagina! Hyaluronic acid is a natural compound that our bodies produce to hydrate different cells in our bodies. Some studies have shown its benefits in vaginal gels by adding back moisture to the vagina for those patients with vaginal dryness who prefer a non-hormonal treatment.

Now if you try those lubes and they don't make a difference, then we can discuss other options like vaginal estrogens. Vaginal estrogen comes in creams – Estrace and Premarin; tablets – Vagifem and Imvexxy; and rings – the Femring and Estring. The good thing about vaginal estrogen is that it works locally mostly, therefore has limited systemic side effects or risks, except the Femring, which is the only one that has both local and systemic effects. Therefore, you will need progesterone to protect your uterine lining if you decide to use the Femring. Supplemental progesterone is not necessary for the other vaginal estrogens, because they only work at the vaginal level. The creams may have a slightly higher risk for systemic effects, but not enough to advise uterine protection using progesterone. The creams are usually prescribed as one to two grams every night for two weeks then two to three times a week for maintenance. Some patients feel that the cream can be too messy. The vaginal tablets have similar instructions of use but aren't messy. The difference between the two types of tablets is that Vagifem is 10 mcg, while Imvexxy, which is the newest, comes in doses of 4 mcg or 10 mcg. You place the rings in your vagina for three months and can still have sex during that time. Once you choose the type that suits you, allow one to three months to notice a significant change. Then you can enjoy sex again!

Urinary symptoms associated with GSM include urgency, pain with urination and recurrent urinary tract infections. Vaginal estrogen may provide some benefit in addressing these symptoms. After ruling out other conditions that may cause these issues, applying vaginal estrogen cream around the urethra can improve these urinary symptoms. Urinary incontinence, which means you will leak urine at different times, is another condition that can occur with aging. Your body can experience changes that certainly involve your pelvic floor muscles that may be associated with prolapse. So, exercise HER! Remember to do your Kegels! Kegel exercises involve actively contracting your vaginal muscles for five seconds, then relaxing your pelvic floor muscles for five seconds. Doing three sets of 10-15 repetitions a day seems to help.

And guess what? Doing Kegels can even improve the intensity of your orgasms! Is that enough motivation? You can also perform Kegels using a Ben Wa ball, a marble-sized ball that you place in your vagina and hold in place for a few seconds to help you exercise those pelvic floor muscles. Please remember to relax those muscles in between contracting them, because too much contraction can cause pelvic pain. If you're doing Kegels and not noticing much improvement, seek guidance from your healthcare provider. Pelvic floor physical therapy is also an option and your provider may direct you in that direction for treatment.

If all else fails, or if you are not a candidate for hormones, vaginal laser therapy is an alternative. Preliminary data suggest that laser technology may offer benefits in treating vaginal atrophy. There certainly has been a craze about "vaginal rejuvenation", which essentially is an umbrella for a host of procedures that alter vaginal or labial tissues for therapeutic or cosmetic purposes. There has been an increase in these procedures since 2014. Vaginal rejuvenation is not the same as vaginal laser therapy. Rejuvenation refers to procedures that alter the size or shape of the vagina and labia, primarily for cosmetic purposes. Vaginal laser therapy focuses on the functional aspects by addressing vaginal dryness, painful sex and urinary symptoms. Its benefits include increasing collagen and elastin production in the vaginal walls, thereby increasing blood supply and hydration, ultimately making sex more comfortable. This procedure is mostly painless. It involves three treatments spaced six weeks apart, where a vaginal probe that releases carbon dioxide laser energy is inserted (other devices may use a different type of thermal energy) for three to five minutes. This procedure is not FDA approved for vaginal symptoms, so you should expect to pay out of pocket for this treatment. In July of 2018, the FDA released a statement that encouraged caution when seeking these types of therapy due to reports of pain and bleeding after the procedure. When used correctly, laser therapy has been shown to be beneficial to women suffering from vaginal atrophy. More data is needed to assess the true safety and effectiveness, especially over a long period of time. But overall, this is a good option for breast cancer survivors or others who have contraindications to hormones. Although controversial, many physicians are using this option off-label to address vaginal atrophy symptoms. Again, having the conversation with your healthcare provider is important to determine your candidacy for this type of procedure.

Words of Affirmation:

I will love and respect "her" because this will enrich my happiness.

8: USE HER OR LOSE HER!

Let's talk about Sex!! The World Health Organization (WHO) describes our sexual health as "a state of physical, emotional, mental and social well-being." This is so true and being mindful of the natural changes your body goes through is an important part of learning how to promote your sexual health throughout the different stages of womanhood.

In the office: A 53-year-old woman comes in for her well woman exam. She asked me, "How old are you, doctor?" I told her my age and then she said, "You just wait until you get into your 50s. You're not gonna want your husband." My response was, "Say what now?!"

I did NOT like the sound of this! So, after I picked my jaw up off the floor, I had to get to the bottom of this! Many women after 40 can experience a decrease in their libido or their sexual desire. These women come into my office looking for a quick fix asking where is my Viagra? Let me speak some truth here.

Remember that book title, Men are from Mars, Women are from Venus? This is real. We are built differently. Men are microwaves – it only takes them a few seconds to get aroused. Women are ovens – it can take us a while to warm up. When I talk about libido, I have to drive to the root, the real cause of this issue. Many times, the issue is above the waist – it's in our heads! And I don't mean this in a bad way. Frankly, if our brains are distracted by other things, sex is the furthest thing from our agendas. Accordingly, I like to ask a few questions to determine where the problem lies:

- Did you lose desire because your vagina feels on fire every time you have sex?
- Did you lose desire when you gained some weight and no longer feel sexy?
- Did you lose desire when you started working two jobs and taking care of three kids?
- Did you lose desire because there are issues in your relationship with your significant other? No attraction, no connection?

- Did you lose desire when you started taking a certain medication?

- Or did you just lose desire and don't know what happened?

These examples display loss of libido in women could be due to many facets. It may not be just one simple issue – it could be multiple. Your job is to self-evaluate and figure out what that might be and my job as the physician is to help you figure this out then discuss some ways of how to rectify it. If you answered yes to one of the questions above, here are some possible reasons:

- If it hurts every time you have sex, eventually you're not going to want to have sex.

- If you don't feel sexy or feel good about yourself, you're not going to want sex.

- If you are overwhelmed with just life and plain tired, you're more interested in sleep than sex.

- If you are having problems in your relationship or losing attraction for your significant other, you're not going to be interested in sex.

- If you are on certain medications, i.e. antidepressants, your libido can be affected negatively.

Libido is also connected to biologic activity regarding certain hormones, like testosterone. So, as you approach menopause or if you're already going through menopause, you will have a decrease in testosterone and that can decrease your libido sometimes. Usually the decrease in testosterone is a more gradual process compared to estrogen levels, but this gradual decrease may not affect every woman's libido in a negative way.

So, what can you do for low libido? Studies have shown testosterone and DHEA have positive effects on your libido. But again, you must determine the etiology of your low libido first. If it's low because sex is painful, then we must address this first. Probably painful due to the vaginal atrophy I discussed in the prior chapter or other reasons that should be investigated such as prolapse or fibroids. So, if we can prevent sex from feeling like "it's adding salt to a wound", according to one of my patients, then there's hope for improving your libido.

We should address vaginal atrophy or dryness first if that is one of your complaints related to sex. If you don't want vaginal estrogen or if you are not a candidate for vaginal estrogen, i.e. breast cancer survivors, then there are some non-estrogen options. Osphemine (Osphena) is a selective estrogen receptor modulator, which acts like estrogen in certain parts of the body. It is an oral tablet taken daily that has been FDA approved for painful intercourse in postmenopausal women. Currently, this drug is not recommended in breast cancer survivors due to its potential hormonal effects on cells in the breast or its potential "estrogen-like" qualities that have a small chance of causing blood clots and a stroke. Keep in mind, hormone replacement therapy has a similar risk regarding blood clots and stroke although this risk is low in healthy individuals. So again, having a conversation with your healthcare provider about your health and determining your candidacy for certain medications is key.

Prasterone (Intrarosa) is another medication that has been FDA approved for painful intercourse. This is a vaginal suppository that you insert every night. It is DHEA that converts to estrogen and testosterone at the vaginal cell level. This medication has become popular, because some studies suggest that DHEA at this level can potentially boost libido. Who wouldn't like that perk!

Let's say you fixed the vaginal dryness with estrogen or with any of the other options and your libido is still not where you want it to be. One natural alternative is Maca, an herb native to the Andes mountains. It is considered an adaptogen, which helps the body adapt to a variety of stressors. It has been used for centuries in other parts of the world to improve sexual function and energy. The evidence is limited, but it appears to have some benefit on the libido of menopausal women. The recommended dose is 2,000-3,000 mg per day.

Testosterone therapy may be an option for you. Testosterone could be given orally and transdermally in compound formulations. Oral formulations are usually not recommended for women due to the side effects. There are also testosterone pellets that can be injected into the hip area, which seem to be more popular in certain areas of the country. Now I would be careful about these pellets due to the fact that these are permanent and could cause a rapid increase of testosterone levels and possibly result in undesirable side effects (hair growth, deepening of voice, acne or an enlarged clitoris). Here is another reason why I may decide to check your hormones, specifically your testosterone levels, to determine your baseline level before starting pellet therapy. If you are considering getting pellets, then I would recommend trying transdermal testosterone first just to see how your body responds to testosterone. If you decide to get the pellets, your testosterone levels should be monitored after implantation. The pellets usually last for about four months, therefore, you would need to get a subsequent dose to maintain effects. Testosterone pellets are usually provided by integrative physicians and/or certain compounding pharmacies. These are not typically provided by your general gynecologist or family medicine physician.

You should also be aware that testosterone therapy in women is not FDA approved, so your insurance may not cover any of these treatments. Now, what about Viagra? The wonder drug for men! What about us women? Well, Flibanserin (Addyi) is the closest to it. It's the only FDA approved medication for hypoactive sexual desire disorder or low libido in women. But, guess what? The studies were only in premenopausal women. So, it is not FDA approved in postmenopausal women. Go figure! Now I'm not saying you can't take it if you are menopausal, but your insurance may not cover it. I know, no fair! But rising studies do show that it works in postmenopausal women as well.

Flibanserin is an oral tablet that you take daily at bedtime and it works at the brain level, as opposed to Viagra, which works at the level of blood vessels in the penis. FYI, Flibanserin has a box warning stating that you can't take this medication and drink alcohol, because the mixture of the two could cause a drop in your blood pressure and syncope. What if we like a glass of wine to get us in the mood? I usually tell patients, to be on the safe side, if you have more than two drinks, don't take your dose that evening. Then you can resume the medication the next night.

Some of you may still ask, "Well can I take Viagra?" Viagra may have some benefit for women who have issues with numbness in the clitoris, because like I said, Viagra works at the level of blood vessels. But, again, this isn't FDA approved, so unlikely to be covered by insurance. The goal with using Viagra would be to improve the stimulation of the clitoris, because we need this tiny organ that God created with the sole purpose of giving US pleasure – there's no other function! It is responsible for 90% of women's orgasms. See, I told you that WE were different. The clitoris has over 8,000 nerve endings, which is twice as many as the penis. Lucky us!

Some women are embarrassed, because they have never achieved an orgasm. A lot of times this could be due to them not being aware of what gets them to climax. So please learn your body and explore what helps you reach your orgasmic pleasure. Even masturbation may be helpful to determine what actually turns you on, because this may change as you get older. Yes, I said masturbation – there's nothing wrong with it! This way you can communicate to your partner what gets your juices flowing! Sex toys are also fun to try, with yourself or even your partner! Again, communication with your partner is key. Introducing a sex toy could spice up a relationship! Some women can also achieve an orgasm through the vagina – oftentimes referred to as the "G spot." This is a small area one-third inside of the top of the vagina that gives much pleasure. Have fun exploring.

Now on to FOREPLAY. Don't forget foreplay! Foreplay is always important, because it can take women a while to warm up. Remember when I said, "women are like ovens"? Foreplay is a must! All this being said, if you haven't figured it out yet, a good sex life is healthy for you. It helps you sleep better, relieves stress and is good exercise. Having an orgasm while losing calories – it's a WIN WIN!

A lot of women are embarrassed by issues they may be having in the bedroom, so they rarely bring it up during appointments with their healthcare provider. Some women are ashamed to admit that it is really affecting their marriage. I encourage you to speak up and this is when being comfortable with your healthcare provider is essential. If you don't feel comfortable, you're not going to talk about it and will suffer in silence. That's not healthy. A good sex life is healthy. So, talking it out may help you on so many levels. I will admit there may be some healthcare providers who also feel uncomfortable about talking about sexual health, so they won't ask you about it. Therefore, you need to be proactive about your sexual health. Ask questions!

Please make your significant other read this and the previous chapter to get an understanding of what could be going on with you as you evolve into your mature self. And spark that fire within to keep the flames going in your relationship, because it's healthy for you!

To all my single ladies, while you're exploring and having your best sex, don't forget to protect yourself. You might not be able to get pregnant (when menopausal), but you can catch something else – Sexually Transmitted Infections (STI)! Good ole' fashion condoms do work. Don't be afraid to ask new partners for their credentials or evidence that they have been tested for STIs in the last six months to one year. The incidence of HIV is rapidly growing in the 50 and over crowd, so protect your vagina and body (your temple) ladies, at ALL times and ages.

Words of Affirmation:

Exercising "her" is essential to my sexual health and consequently improving my overall well-being.

9: THE OTHER WOMAN…

"Doctor, I have a very short fuse."

"Doctor, I sometimes cry, and I don't know why."

"Doctor, my husband is complaining I'm very moody, but I can't control it."

"Doctor, I can't remember things like I used to."

These are all statements that I have heard in my office from women who are going through perimenopause or menopause. Mental health can greatly be affected by menopause. A lot of women feel like they are on an emotional roller coaster and they really want to get off. PMS can also worsen when you're perimenopausal. Women report that they are becoming a person that they do not recognize, hence "the OTHER woman." Menopause can generate depression and/or anxiety. It can also resurrect or worsen depression and anxiety if you've been diagnosed with them in the past.

Naturally, depending on your history, I would start discussing non-prescription options with you. First, avoid potential triggers that can exacerbate mental health issues like caffeine and alcohol, which can potentially intensify anxiety. Here I go trying to get rid of your glass of wine again, but everything must be used in moderation, if at all, based on your symptoms.

Secondly, discuss your symptoms with your physician and ensure there are no underlying medical conditions that could cause anxiety, like a thyroid disorder. Thirdly, again, exercise is very important. The release of endorphins during exercise can certainly create a sense of calm. I recommend exercising at least five days per week, 30-45 minutes per day. And pick an activity you like to do. Personally, I do NOT like running on a treadmill. I had to force myself to do it and it wasn't enjoyable. I used to drag myself downstairs to my basement to get on the treadmill. After trying different things, I've realized that I enjoy spinning and look forward to exercising now.

Finally, improving your nutrition is always a plus. Some data has shown deficiency in the B vitamins, specifically B6, could be linked to mood disorders. Vitamin B6 and omega-3 fatty acids can be helpful in improving mood. Dietary sources of Vitamin B6 are chickpeas, yellowfin tuna and salmon. B6 supplementation should not exceed 100 mg daily, because it could lead to neurologic issues. Deficiency in omega-3 fatty acids could be related to increased anxiety. Dietary sources of omega-3 could be found in a variety of fish (sardines, tuna and salmon), chia seeds and flaxseeds. Or you could take fish oil supplements daily.

Ashwagandha is an Indian herb that may have some calming properties, potentially helpful in relieving stress. Evening Primrose oil and Vitamin E may potentially help with mood symptoms too. St. John's Wort is a botanical that has been used to alleviate depression and the suggested dosage is 300 mg, three times per day. Although the evidence is limited, St. John's Wort can be taken by itself or in combination with other herbs, like black cohosh, to relieve depression and/or mood swings. Caution should be used when combining it with prescription medications, because it could interfere with the metabolism of certain medications.

Serenol is a new supplement on the market, launched in the U.S. in 2015. It is a blend of Swedish pollen extract, chromium picolinate and royal jelly, which is a substance created by honeybees (not recommended if you are allergic to bees). It has been shown to help the emotional symptoms of PMS, including irritability, mood swings and food cravings.

Sleep! Make sure you are getting enough sleep, because the lack of sleep can lead to fatigue and short tempers. Yoga and/or meditation can be good for your spirit. I highly recommend making this part of your routine. I try to recommend these practices to all of my patients, because it can make a big difference in mood and attitude throughout the menopausal process. Essential oils, like lavender, neroli and peppermint, can also be helpful in improving your overall mood.

It is important to discuss this with your healthcare provider and decide what are some good options for you. Like I stated before, "Talk it Out!" More importantly, don't be afraid to seek counseling with a psychologist or a psychiatrist if necessary. Having an objective ear to listen to your thoughts and concerns can be therapeutic.

If you try natural options and don't notice any real improvement or if you wanted to add a medication to the natural alternatives, there are plenty of antidepressant and anti-anxiety medications that could be prescribed. And don't be fearful about going this route. Many women are hesitant about starting medication, because they fear the stigma of being on antidepressant or antianxiety drugs. A lot of times family or your culture deter you from trying this option and you try to avoid being judged or labeled as "weak".

Taking a medication to improve your mental health does NOT make you weak. Not taking it when you need it, can be detrimental! Negative thinking does NOT produce positive outcomes. Be proactive and do what you need to do to improve your mental health. Even if you start these types of medications, this doesn't mean you have to be on it forever. But if you must, so be it. If you are symptom free for 6-12 months, you can consider weaning yourself off the medication but again discuss it with your healthcare provider as you make this decision.

Common antidepressants are Fluoxetine (Prozac), Sertraline (Zoloft), Citalopram (Celexa), Paroxetine (Paxil) and Buproprion (Wellbutrin). These medications could also be used to treat an anxiety component. Escitalopram (Lexapro) and Duloxetine (Cymbalta) can treat both depression and anxiety. Common antianxiety medication is Venlafaxine (Effexor). Other anti-anxiety medications that are short-acting are Alprazolam (Xanax) and Lorazepam (Ativan), but these could be habit-forming.

Do they have side effects? Yes. The biggest complaints are weight gain and sexual dysfunction. Buproprion seems to be the only one that has the least risk of weight gain and sexual dysfunction. In fact, its mechanism of action can cause the complete opposite. You also need to consider how much of the weight gain and/or sexual dysfunction is due to the actual depression or the medication. A good conversation with your healthcare provider can lead to an option that is best for you.

You may tell your doctor, "I feel like my brain is in a fog" or "I don't remember things anymore. Even the simplest of things and my mind draws a blank. This is not like me!"

Brain fog and the inability to remember things is very real in menopause but is usually temporary. Some data suggest taking the Chinese herb gingko biloba, may be helpful with these symptoms. Researchers believe that it increases circulation in the brain, which ultimately improves cognitive function.

Some women come into my office crying, because they just don't recognize themselves. They've become a different woman – the OTHER woman. Things are happening to their mind and bodies beyond their control. It can be disheartening and scary. Just remember, you will get through it. Hopefully, it is all temporary. I think it's helpful for you to know that 1) these mental changes are real and 2) you are not alone, so resist the feelings of isolation and frustration.

Discussions with your provider will determine if starting a prescribed medication is necessary. Be sure to review your medical conditions, other medications/supplements you're taking and potential side effects of the medications.

These are the times when you need to make YOUR TIME a priority. Making time for ourselves is so difficult when we're running around doing things for others or just worrying about them. It really helps our mental health. This could be time to get a massage or a pedicure, sit alone and read a book or do ANYTHING that YOU want to do. We all make excuses that "there just isn't enough time for me." Well, guess what? If you don't make YOUR time a priority, eventually you won't be well, and you won't be able to take care of anyone. You must pencil yourself onto your calendar. If you can cut back some work hours, do it! Don't be afraid to use your power of saying "No" to things that may interfere with YOUR time. The work-life balance is SO important for our mental state.

In 2016, I made a very difficult decision to stop doing Obstetrics, which is what I loved the most about my profession. But my work schedule, being a mommy to three kids and a wife no longer fit together nicely into my "perfect" world. Being pulled in so many directions was mentally draining, and it was also raising my blood pressure, so I had to make some changes. I was also lucky to have a primary care physician who strongly encouraged me to make time for myself. And now she is happy that I finally listened because I no longer need that blood pressure medicine. It was very difficult for me to step back and unload some of my responsibilities because, you know as women, we feel we should be able to do it ALL. Well, we CAN, but do we really WANT to, or do we HAVE to?

I also found journaling to be helpful to my mental well-being, so I started doing it at least three times per week. Get yourself a journal to write down your thoughts and concerns if you don't already have one. Personally, I feel that this a good outlet that allows you to write down your positive and negative feelings/thoughts. You should try to write about things that you are grateful for. Challenge yourself to focus on positive things in your life. Positive thinking creates positive results and experiences. So instead of being the "other" woman, be the woman that is evolving and working toward being the best version of herself.

Words of Affirmation:

We are not perfect human beings, nor do we have to pretend to be. But it is necessary for us to be the best version of ourselves we can be. - Anonymous

10: A POTPOURRI OF OTHER SYMPTOMS

There are other symptoms that I didn't dedicate a whole chapter to, but that certainly can be a part of the perimenopause/menopause experience:

• Weight gain are two words we hate hearing, right? You can gain weight mostly around your midsection and it can be very annoying. Despite no change in diet nor exercise, you still gain weight. Well, you can't cut the same corners you could when you were younger, like eating large portions, unhealthy snacking, happy hour (alcohol=calories) and little to no exercise. Aging does affect your metabolism. So you must eat healthy AND exercise, to lose the weight and maintain a healthy weight. You should eat mindfully and eat healthy snacks under 200 calories. A small portion of dark chocolate (one-inch flat square) can be a healthy and happy treat. Portion control is one of the biggest issues contributing to weight gain. You don't have to eat until you're full. We can teach ourselves to be satisfied with less. (I'm still working on this!).

- Insomnia is difficulty falling asleep, staying asleep or waking up too early in the morning. Getting adequate sleep can help with weight loss. Good sleep hygiene requires seven to eight hours of sleep. (I think the last time I got this much sleep, I was in high school.) You should set a regular schedule if possible, avoid daytime naps, control your sleep environment, (proper lighting, limited noise or soothing music, turn off the electronics and a comfortable room temperature), regular exercise, (don't forget good sex), good eating habits, (avoid potential stimulants before bed like caffeine, smoking or alcohol) and manage stress (yoga and meditation may help). Calming teas, like chamomile and passion flower, can be useful. If you still need assistance after changing some habits, you can try 2 mg prolonged release of melatonin two hours before bedtime. Short-acting melatonin may not work as well. Taking 600 mg of valerian root extract per day is another option. There are prescribed medications that are available, such as Ambien, but this could be habit-forming or result in the feeling of a hangover the following morning. Antidepressants that have sedating effects, like Trazadone, Serzone or Remeron could also be prescribed.

- Migraines or headaches can increase in frequency. I usually recommend taking 300-600 mg of a magnesium supplement per day if other medical conditions have been ruled out.

- Female pattern hair loss or thinning can occur on the crown and temples. A workup is necessary to exclude systemic causes of hair loss such as thyroid disease. The FDA-approved Minoxidil, a topical foam applied daily, can possibly help some women with mild hair loss by preventing any further hair loss. The supplement Biotin can also be supportive during this process.

- Acne and/or excess hair growth can occur due to the decline in estrogen relative to the number of circulating androgens like testosterone. Therefore, the treatment goal is to decrease the number of circulating androgens. Hormones could be used to counteract this imbalance. Spironolactone is a medication that has anti-androgen effects that can be helpful in decreasing acne, as well as hair growth. Cosmetic hair removal strategies, like laser hair removal or electrolysis, are also options to consider for excess hair growth. Determining a good skin care regimen is also important for your skin, in addition to determining if certain triggers, like stress or high sugar foods, contribute to your acne breakouts. Also, if you are on birth control, certain progestins can worsen your acne; specifically, those containing etonogestrel or levonorgestrel. You may seek assistance from a dermatologist for other strategies for acne prevention such as isotretinoin.

- Breast pain or tenderness is common. The fluctuation of hormones can cause this. Caffeine can also play a big role, so cutting caffeine intake may be helpful. Evening primrose oil and vitamin E have also been shown to improve breast pain.

Although breast pain can be common, please report these new symptoms to your healthcare provider to get a proper evaluation.

- Joint pain can be new complaint. Some research suggests benefits from taking 1500 mg of glucosamine per day, 1 g of chondroitin per day or 2 g of turmeric per day. Use caution with turmeric, because it can thin your blood causing easy bruising.

- Dry skin and/or dry eyes could occur, your vagina is not the only one that dries out. Ensure you are adequately hydrated. Drinking plenty of water is always good. Find good moisturizing lotions/oils for the skin. Taking fish oil tablets seem to help with dry eyes.

Nutrition activates hormones and signaling pathways in the gut, which can affect your appetite, sleep, energy, cognitive function and mood. This reminds us that adequate nutrition plays a role in the balance of hormones and overall well-being. Taking a probiotic daily can also be helpful in regulating the metabolism in your gut. Probiotics with lactobacillus can also help with vaginal health and decrease the frequency of vaginal infections.

Before starting any supplements, please contact your healthcare provider to determine if it's okay to try them along with other medications you may be taking. Your health care provider may want to check certain laboratory studies before starting supplements to determine any deficiencies. Also, all the medications and/or supplements that I mention in this book are FOR YOUR INFORMATION only. I have no financial ties to any of them. My goal again is to make you are aware of your options so you can make an informed decision about your health. Please keep in mind that this complex world of menopause is still being studied and I'm sure there will be more medications that become available after this book is in your hands.

Words of Affirmation:

God made me a woman because HE knew I could handle this journey.

11: LIVING YOUR BEST LIFE

I can't finish this book without discussing some preventive strategies you need to follow as you approach menopause. I can't stress enough that exercise and eating healthy are important. Cardiovascular disease is the leading cause of death in women, so protect your heart. Your cholesterol levels can change during menopause, predisposing you to high cholesterol and high blood pressure. Knowing your family history is also important, because you can do everything you can to be healthy, but if it's in your genes, it's harder to avoid. So be proactive before it catches up to you.

Eat the rainbow! Eat lots of fruits and vegetables. You need 30 g of fiber to maintain good cholesterol. You need to exercise at least for 30 minutes, at least five days per week. Find an exercise that you like. At first, I dreaded exercise and didn't do much in the beginning of my journey to a healthy lifestyle. But like I said before, once I made spinning my favorite exercise, I look forward to exercising to decrease some stress. Again, you must find something that you like to do. Something that allows you to clear your mind and destress. You don't have to jump straight into 30 minutes for five days. You can start off slowly, then work your way to that goal. I always remind my patients that you must make attainable goals when you begin your wellness journey. If you don't, you're setting yourself up for failure. Remember, it is a lifestyle change, not a quick fix!

Routine screening is also important to your journey to good health and wellness. A 69-year-old patient said me, "Doctor, I've been getting pap smears every year since I can remember, but now that I'm older, I don't need them every year. So, you don't care if I get cancer?" I explained how this is partly true. Of course, I care, but it's just not necessary, especially if you are considered low-risk. There are guidelines that gynecologists follow to determine when a patient needs a pap smear. Before I explain the appropriate pap smear schedule, let's review Human Papilloma Virus (HPV). HPV is a sexually transmitted virus that is present in about 90% of the population that engage in sexual activity. Checking your HPV status usually starts at age 30, however, may be obtained sooner if you have an abnormal pap smear. HPV is checked every 3 years with your pap smear. Some gynecologists may use a five-year schedule. The American College of Obstetrics & Gynecology (ACOG) recommends HPV status checks every three to five years based on prior research. A pap smear is a screening test for cervical cancer and HPV is the virus that causes cervical cancer as well as anal and throat cancer. Therefore, pap with HPV is done every three years in my office up to the ages of 65-70. ACOG states you can stop having pap smears after age 65, but again, only if you qualify to be in the low-risk population. Your risk of cervical cancer at this age is quite low. But this does NOT mean that you should see your gynecologist or family care physician every three years. You still should see us annually to get your pelvic and breast exams and to assess your overall health on a regular basis. Although, with Medicare, you are advised to see the gynecologist every other year, again, only if you are considered to be low-risk. After the age of 80, I typically advise annual pelvic exams are no longer necessary if you are at low risk for gynecologic cancer, especially if you've already had a hysterectomy and/or removal of your ovaries. But this a personal decision, some women still choose to come annually and that is okay.

There has been conflicting data on mammogram schedules. I typically go by the ACOG guidelines and your typical low-risk patient should start mammograms at age 40. If you are high-risk, (significant family history, known presence of breast cancer gene), then you should get them sooner in addition to considering additional genetic testing. If there isn't any family history, you have the option of getting a mammogram every other year up to age 50. Then after 50, annually. There is also controversy about self-breast exams and if patients should still do them. I still recommend them monthly. A lot of breast cancers are found by the patient.

Bone density scans usually start at age 65 but begin sooner if you have certain risk factors (early or premature menopause, family history of osteoporosis, history of fracture from low-impact trauma over the age of 50, smoking, a very thin body build or chronic steroid use). Bone loss rapidly increases after age 30 and well into the start of menopause. Osteoporosis is a disease characterized by low bone mass and deterioration of bone, which increases the risk for fractures. To decrease your risk, don't forget to take your calcium and vitamin D. You need 1200 mg of Calcium and at least 1000 IU of vitamin D3 daily. Don't forget your weight bearing exercises like walking, aerobics and weight training. A colonoscopy screens for colorectal cancer and is usually due at age 50, but sooner if you have a positive family history of colon cancer.

Amidst these preventive goals, find the **time** for YOU. Your **top priorities** should be maintaining **good health** and scheduling **time** to show yourself some love. Doing what is necessary to maintain good health like eating healthy, exercise and meditation. And don't forget good sex is very important to your health. Your preventive exams should be on a regular basis. These steps all require making the time to do them, invest in yourself. Once again, make time for yourself to just do you. Get a massage, read a good book or take a short vacation. As women, we get caught up in taking care of everybody else around us but forget about ourselves. You are important too and you're worth it!

Every woman goes through menopause in some shape or fashion. Some may cruise through it and others hit many bumps along the way. Just remember, you ALL will get through it no matter what. Don't fight it, it's natural. Remember change can be good, although it can be uncomfortable. You are evolving into an enhanced you. It's not the menopausal takeover, but the menopausal makeover. If you weren't taking good care of yourself before, then NOW is the time. If you were taking good care of yourself, then you may have to do some things differently to maintain wellness. Through it all, be informed, so that you can make the right decision for YOU. Your mind, body and spirit depend on it! And through it all, stand strong in your truth saying, "I am living my best life loving me, myself and "her!"

Words of Affirmation:

Don't compare your life to others. There's no comparison between the sun and the moon. They shine when it's their time. -womenworking.com

Embrace your own unique shine!!

Made in the USA
Middletown, DE
20 April 2019